The Complete 0 Point Food List

Fuel Your Body Right: The Ultimate Zero-Point Food Compendium for Sustainable Nutrition

McDonnell B. Young

Table of Contents

Introduction

Emma sat at her kitchen table, flipping through a stack of cookbooks, feeling overwhelmed. After years of struggling with her weight and health issues, she had decided to make a change. The constant cycle of fad diets and confusing nutritional advice left her disheartened. She needed a solution that was simple, effective, and sustainable.

One evening, while scrolling through online reviews for yet another diet guide, Emma came across "The Complete 0 Point Food List." The title piqued her curiosity. It promised a straightforward approach to eating without the need for complex calculations or restrictive rules. The guide boasted a comprehensive list of foods that had zero points—foods that could be enjoyed freely without guilt or concern over calorie counts.

Emma decided to give it a chance. The next day, her copy arrived. As she flipped through the pages, she felt a sense of excitement. The guide was more than just a list; it was a complete resource. It began with a clear explanation of what 0 point foods were and why they were beneficial. This was followed by an easy-to-navigate section detailing which vegetables, fruits, proteins, and dairy products were included in the 0 point category. Emma appreciated the organized layout, which made it simple to find information quickly.

The guide didn't stop at listing foods. It provided practical advice on how to incorporate them into daily meals. With sample meal plans for breakfast, lunch, dinner, and snacks, Emma could easily see how to use these foods in a variety of delicious, satisfying ways. The recipe section included creative and tasty ideas for salads, soups, and smoothies, which inspired her to experiment in the kitchen.

One of the most helpful aspects was the section on foods to avoid. Emma learned which items could sabotage her progress and why. This allowed her to make informed choices when shopping and dining out, reducing the temptation to stray from her new path.

The guide also offered practical tips for success, including meal prep strategies, shopping advice, and portion control techniques. Emma felt empowered by these insights, knowing she had the tools to maintain her new eating habits. The FAQs section addressed common concerns and provided solutions to potential challenges, which reassured her that she was not alone in her journey.

As Emma implemented the guide's recommendations, she noticed significant changes. Her energy levels improved, and she began to see gradual, sustainable weight loss. Meals were no longer a source of stress but a joyful experience. The simple approach of the 0 point foods allowed her to enjoy a variety of flavors without the need for meticulous tracking or deprivation.

"The Complete 0 Point Food List" became more than just a book for Emma; it was a trusted companion in her journey towards better health. She appreciated how the guide made healthy eating accessible and enjoyable, proving that simplicity and balance could lead to lasting success.

If you're like Emma, feeling overwhelmed by complicated diets and endless restrictions, "The Complete 0 Point Food List" is the guide you need. It's a user-friendly resource that demystifies healthy eating, making it achievable and satisfying. With this guide, you can take the first step towards a healthier, more fulfilling lifestyle, just like Emma did.

Overview of 0 Point Foods

In the realm of nutrition and dietary management, 0 point foods offer a distinctive advantage, particularly for those seeking simplicity in their eating plans. These foods are essentially those that have minimal to no impact on overall caloric intake, making them ideal for individuals aiming to maintain or lose weight while still enjoying a satisfying range of options. The concept of 0 point foods is designed to facilitate easier tracking and planning of meals, allowing for greater flexibility and variety in one's diet without the constant need to calculate points or calories.

One of the primary benefits of 0 point foods lies in their ability to satiate hunger without contributing significantly to daily caloric goals. This means that individuals can eat these foods freely, which can be especially helpful for those who struggle with portion control or frequent cravings. By focusing on these low-calorie, nutrient-dense options, individuals can manage their intake more effectively and reduce the likelihood of feeling deprived or restricted.

The Complete 0 Point Food List provides a comprehensive overview of these advantageous foods, categorizing them into various groups such as vegetables, fruits, proteins, and dairy products. Vegetables, for instance, form a cornerstone of the 0 point category, given their high fiber content and low energy density. These foods not only help in feeling full but also contribute essential vitamins and minerals necessary for overall health. Leafy greens, cruciferous vegetables, and root vegetables are just a few examples that appear frequently in this category.

Fruits also play a significant role in the 0 point food list, with many options being naturally low in calories and high in water content. Berries, citrus fruits, and melons are particularly noted for their ability to provide a sweet treat without added sugars or excessive calories. These fruits are not only enjoyable but also packed with antioxidants and other beneficial compounds that support long-term wellness.

Proteins included in the 0 point list offer a substantial benefit for those looking to build muscle or maintain energy levels while managing calorie intake. Lean poultry, fish, and plant-based options like tofu are featured as prime examples. These protein sources are essential for muscle repair and growth, and their low calorie content ensures that they fit seamlessly into a balanced eating plan without contributing to weight gain.

Dairy and dairy alternatives also make an appearance on the 0 point list, with non-fat or low-fat options providing necessary calcium and protein. Products such as skim milk and unsweetened almond milk are highlighted for their minimal caloric content while still delivering essential nutrients. This inclusion supports a well-rounded diet that can cater to various dietary preferences and restrictions.

The list is not just about what to include but also what to avoid. By outlining which foods are better left off the 0 point list, individuals are guided towards making healthier choices that align with their goals. Foods high in added sugars, refined grains, and unhealthy fats are carefully omitted to prevent potential setbacks in one's dietary journey.

Overall, "The Complete 0 Point Food List" serves as a valuable tool for anyone seeking a straightforward approach to healthier eating. By focusing on foods that offer maximum satiety with minimal caloric impact, the guide simplifies the process of making beneficial dietary choices. This approach not only supports weight management but also fosters a sustainable and enjoyable eating experience.

Benefits of 0 Point Foods

The concept of 0 point foods offers a transformative approach to healthy eating, making it easier for individuals to manage their weight and overall health. By incorporating foods that are assigned zero points into daily meals, people can enjoy a wide range of nutritious options without the need for restrictive calorie counting or portion control. This system simplifies the dietary process, allowing individuals to focus on making healthier choices without feeling deprived.

One of the primary benefits of 0 point foods is their contribution to a balanced diet. These foods are typically rich in essential nutrients such as vitamins, minerals, and fiber while being low in calories and unhealthy fats. By consuming these nutrient-dense options, individuals can meet their nutritional needs effectively while avoiding excess calories that contribute to weight gain. This balance promotes overall health and supports the body's functions more efficiently.

Additionally, 0 point foods are known for their ability to promote satiety and reduce hunger. Foods like leafy greens, fruits, and lean proteins can help individuals feel full longer, which is crucial for managing appetite and preventing overeating. This natural satiety helps individuals stay on track with their health goals by reducing the likelihood of snacking on high-calorie, less nutritious options between meals.

The flexibility of 0 point foods also enhances their appeal. Since these foods can be consumed freely, individuals have the freedom to create diverse and satisfying meals. This flexibility fosters a positive relationship with food, as people are not restricted to monotonous or bland diets. Instead, they can explore various recipes and meal ideas that incorporate a wide range of 0 point foods, keeping meals interesting and enjoyable.

Another significant advantage of 0 point foods is their role in supporting long-term dietary adherence. When people do not feel restricted by their food choices, they are more likely to stick with a healthy eating plan. The absence of stringent rules makes the diet more sustainable, as individuals can integrate 0 point foods into their lives without feeling like they are missing out or constantly battling cravings.

Moreover, incorporating 0 point foods can lead to positive lifestyle changes beyond just diet. As people become more mindful of their food choices and embrace a healthier eating pattern, they may also experience increased energy levels, improved mood, and better overall well-being. These improvements can motivate continued commitment to a healthier lifestyle and encourage further positive changes.

In essence, the benefits of 0 point foods extend beyond mere weight management. They support a holistic approach to health by providing a foundation for balanced nutrition, promoting satiety, and enhancing the overall enjoyment of eating. This approach allows individuals to achieve their health goals while fostering a positive and sustainable relationship with food.

How to Use This Guide

Using "The Complete 0 Point Food List" effectively involves understanding how to integrate its content into your daily routine to achieve optimal results. Begin by familiarizing yourself with the concept of 0 point foods, which are those that contribute no points to your daily intake, allowing you to consume them freely. These foods are carefully selected for their nutritional value and low caloric density, making them ideal for promoting weight management and overall health.

Start by exploring the detailed list of 0 point foods provided in the guide. This list includes a wide variety of vegetables, fruits, proteins, and dairy alternatives. Pay attention to the categories and types of foods included, as these will form the basis of your meals. Incorporating these foods into your diet will help you stay full and satisfied while maintaining a healthy caloric balance.

Next, use the guide's sample meal plans as a starting point for creating your own. These plans offer practical examples of how to combine 0 point foods into balanced meals for breakfast, lunch, dinner, and snacks. Feel free to adapt these meal ideas based on your personal preferences and dietary needs. The guide's meal plans are designed to be flexible, providing a framework that you can modify as you discover what works best for you.

The recipe section of the guide is a valuable resource for adding variety to your meals. Explore the recipes for salads, soups, and smoothies that feature 0 point foods. These recipes are designed to be both nutritious and flavorful, making it easier to stick to your eating plan. Try experimenting with these recipes and adjust the ingredients to suit your taste while ensuring you adhere to the 0 point guidelines.

When shopping for groceries, use the guide's recommendations to make informed choices. The list of foods to avoid is equally important as the list of foods to eat. By steering clear of high-calorie, high-fat, and processed items, you can better manage your dietary intake and prevent setbacks. This proactive approach to grocery shopping will help you maintain a healthier pantry and make more mindful food choices.

Meal prep and planning are crucial aspects of successfully using this guide. The guide provides tips on how to prepare and store meals in advance, which can save you time and make it easier to stick to your plan. Plan your meals for the week, prepare ingredients ahead of time, and create a routine that fits your lifestyle. This organization will help you stay on track and make healthier choices more consistently.

Finally, refer to the FAQs section for guidance on any questions or challenges that arise as you use the guide. This section offers practical solutions to common issues and provides reassurance as you navigate your new eating plan. Embracing the tips and strategies outlined in the guide will support your journey towards better health, making the process of adopting 0 point foods a rewarding and manageable experience.

Chapter 1: Foods to Eat

Vegetables

Here is a detailed table on "Vegetables" from "The Complete 0 Point Food List," including ingredient details, instructions, nutritional information, serving size, and cooking time:

Vegetable	Ingredients	Instructions	Nutritional Information	Serving Size	Cooking Time
Spinach	Fresh spinach leaves	Wash thoroughly. Use raw in salads or lightly sauté for 2-3	7 calories, 1g protein, 1g carbs, 0g fat	1 cup cooked	2-3 minutes

		minutes.			
Kale	Fresh kale leaves	Wash and remove stems. Sauté for 3-4 minutes or use in salads.	33 calories, 2g protein, 6g carbs, 0.5g fat	1 cup cooked	3-4 minutes
Broccoli	Fresh broccoli florets	Steam or boil for 5-7 minutes. Can also be roasted.	55 calories, 4g protein, 11g carbs, 0.6g fat	1 cup cooked	5-7 minutes
Cauliflower	Fresh cauliflower florets	Steam, boil, or roast for 6-8	25 calories, 2g protein, 5g	1 cup cooked	6-8 minutes

		minutes .	carbs, 0.1g fat		
Bell Peppers	Fresh bell peppers	Slice and eat raw or sauté for 4-5 minutes .	31 calories, 1g protein, 7g carbs, 0.3g fat	1 cup cooked	4-5 minutes
Cucum bers	Fresh cucum bers	Peel and slice. Eat raw or add to salads.	16 calories, 1g protein, 4g carbs, 0g fat	1 cup sliced	None
Zucchi ni	Fresh zucchin i slices	Sauté for 4-5 minutes or roast for 10-15 minutes .	17 calories, 1g protein, 3g carbs, 0.3g fat	1 cup cooked	4-5 minutes

Green Beans	Fresh green beans	Steam or boil for 4-6 minutes. Can be sautéed as well.	31 calories, 2g protein, 7g carbs, 0.1g fat	1 cup cooked	4-6 minutes
Asparagus	Fresh asparagus spears	Steam, boil, or roast for 4-6 minutes.	20 calories, 2g protein, 4g carbs, 0.2g fat	1 cup cooked	4-6 minutes
Brussels Sprouts	Fresh Brussels sprouts	Steam or roast for 6-8 minutes.	38 calories, 3g protein, 8g carbs, 0.3g fat	1 cup cooked	6-8 minutes

Tomatoes	Fresh tomatoes	Eat raw or cook for 5 minutes. Can be used in salads or sauces.	22 calories, 1g protein, 5g carbs, 0.2g fat	1 cup cooked	5 minutes
Mushrooms	Fresh mushrooms	Sauté for 5-7 minutes. Can be added to salads or other dishes.	15 calories, 2g protein, 2g carbs, 0.2g fat	1 cup cooked	5-7 minutes
Carrots	Fresh carrots	Eat raw or cook for 5-7 minutes. Can	41 calories, 1g protein, 10g	1 cup cooked	5-7 minutes

		be steamed or roasted.	carbs, 0.2g fat		
Celery	Fresh celery stalks	Eat raw or cook for 5 minutes . Can be added to salads and soups.	16 calories, 1g protein, 3g carbs, 0.2g fat	1 cup sliced	5 minutes
Beets	Fresh beets	Roast for 45-60 minutes or boil for 30-40 minutes .	43 calories, 2g protein, 10g carbs, 0.2g fat	1 cup cooked	45-60 minutes

This table provides a comprehensive overview of various vegetables included in "The Complete 0 Point Food List," detailing their preparation, nutritional content, serving sizes, and cooking times.

Fruits

Here is a detailed and comprehensive table about fruits in relation to "The Complete 0 Point Food List," including ingredients, instructions, nutritional information, serving size, and cooking time:

Fruit	Ingredient	Instructions	Nutritional Information (per serving)	Serving Size	Cooking Time
Apple	1 medium apple	Wash and slice. Eat raw or add to salads.	Calories: 95, Carbs: 25g, Fiber: 4g, Sugar: 19g	1 medium apple	None
Orange	1 medium	Peel and segmen	Calories: 62, Carbs:	1 medium	None

	m orange	t. Eat raw or add to fruit salads.	15g, Fiber: 3g, Sugar: 12g	m orange	
Strawb erries	1 cup sliced strawbe rries	Wash and slice. Eat raw or add to yogurt or salads.	Calories : 49, Carbs: 12g, Fiber: 3g, Sugar: 7g	1 cup	None
Bluebe rries	1 cup fresh blueber ries	Wash and eat raw. Can be added to cereals or yogurt.	Calories : 84, Carbs: 21g, Fiber: 4g, Sugar: 15g	1 cup	None

Raspbe rries	1 cup fresh raspber ries	Wash and eat raw. Can be added to smooth ies or desserts.	Calories : 65, Carbs: 15g, Fiber: 8g, Sugar: 5g	1 cup	None
Water melon	2 cups diced waterm elon	Wash and cube. Eat raw or add to fruit salads.	Calories : 60, Carbs: 15g, Fiber: 0.6g, Sugar: 9g	2 cups	None
Cantal oupe	1 cup diced cantalo upe	Wash and cube. Eat raw or add to fruit salads.	Calories : 54, Carbs: 14g, Fiber: 1.4g, Sugar: 13g	1 cup	None

Honey dew	1 cup diced honeyd ew	Wash and cube. Eat raw or add to fruit salads.	Calories : 61, Carbs: 16g, Fiber: 0.8g, Sugar: 14g	1 cup	None
Peach	1 mediu m peach	Wash and slice. Eat raw or add to yogurt.	Calories : 59, Carbs: 15g, Fiber: 2g, Sugar: 13g	1 mediu m peach	None
Pear	1 mediu m pear	Wash and slice. Eat raw or add to salads.	Calories : 96, Carbs: 26g, Fiber: 5g, Sugar: 17g	1 mediu m pear	None

Grapes	1 cup grapes	Wash and eat raw. Can be frozen for a cool snack.	Calories: 62, Carbs: 16g, Fiber: 1g, Sugar: 16g	1 cup	None
Kiwi	1 medium kiwi	Peel and slice. Eat raw or add to fruit salads.	Calories: 42, Carbs: 10g, Fiber: 2g, Sugar: 7g	1 medium kiwi	None
Plum	1 medium plum	Wash and slice. Eat raw or add to salads.	Calories: 30, Carbs: 8g, Fiber: 1g, Sugar: 6g	1 medium plum	None

Pineap ple	1 cup diced pineapp le	Peel, core, and cube. Eat raw or add to smooth ies.	Calories : 82, Carbs: 22g, Fiber: 2g, Sugar: 16g	1 cup	None
Mango	1 cup diced mango	Peel and cube. Eat raw or add to salsas.	Calories : 99, Carbs: 25g, Fiber: 3g, Sugar: 23g	1 cup	None

This table provides a concise overview of various fruits that are part of "The Complete 0 Point Food List," highlighting how they can be used, their nutritional benefits, and basic preparation methods.

Proteins

Here is a detailed and comprehensive table for "Proteins" in relation to "The Complete 0 Point Food List":

Protein	Ingredients	Instructions	Nutritional Information (per serving)	Serving Size	Cooking Time
Chicken Breast	Skinless chicken breast	Grill, bake, or sauté until cooked through.	Calories: 165, Protein: 31g, Fat: 3.6g	4 oz	20-30 minutes
Turkey Breast	Skinless turkey breast	Roast or grill until internal temperature	Calories: 135, Protein: 30g, Fat: 1g	4 oz	25-35 minutes

		reaches 165°F.			
Cod	Fresh or frozen cod	Bake or poach until fish flakes easily with a fork.	Calories : 90, Protein: 20g, Fat: 0.7g	4 oz	15-20 minutes
Tilapia	Fresh or frozen tilapia	Pan-fry, bake, or grill until fish is opaque and flakes.	Calories : 111, Protein: 23g, Fat: 2.3g	4 oz	10-15 minutes
Salmon	Fresh or frozen salmon	Bake, grill, or pan-sear until fish is cooked	Calories : 206, Protein: 22g, Fat: 13g	4 oz	15-20 minutes

		through .			
Egg Whites	Egg whites	Scramble or cook in a non-stick pan.	Calories: 17, Protein: 3.6g, Fat: 0g	1/4 cup	5 minutes
Tofu	Firm tofu	Sauté, grill, or bake until golden and crispy.	Calories: 94, Protein: 10g, Fat: 5g	4 oz	10-20 minutes
Tempeh	Tempeh	Sauté, grill, or bake until golden brown.	Calories: 192, Protein: 19g, Fat: 11g	4 oz	10-15 minutes

Greek Yogurt (Non-F at)	Non-fat Greek yogurt	Eat as is or use in recipes.	Calories : 80, Protein: 15g, Fat: 0g	1 cup	No cooking needed
Skim Milk	Skim milk	Drink or use in cooking and baking.	Calories : 83, Protein: 8g, Fat: 0.2g	1 cup	No cooking needed
Cottage Cheese (Low-F at)	Low-fat cottage cheese	Eat as is or add to dishes.	Calories : 90, Protein: 11g, Fat: 1g	1/2 cup	No cooking needed
Edama me	Shelled edama me	Steam or boil until tender.	Calories : 120, Protein: 11g, Fat: 5g	1/2 cup	5-10 minutes
Lentils	Dried lentils	Cook in water or	Calories : 115,	1/2 cup cooked	20-30 minutes

		broth until tender.	Protein: 9g, Fat: 0.4g		
Black Beans	Canned or cooked black beans	Rinse and use in recipes.	Calories: 114, Protein: 8g, Fat: 0.5g	1/2 cup cooked	10 minutes (canned)
Chickp eas	Canned or cooked chickpe as	Rinse and use in recipes.	Calories: 134, Protein: 7g, Fat: 2g	1/2 cup cooked	10 minutes (canned)

This table provides an overview of various 0 point proteins, including their preparation methods, nutritional content, serving sizes, and cooking times, helping you make informed choices and streamline your meal planning.

Dairy and Dairy Alternatives

Here is a detailed and comprehensive table for "Dairy and Dairy Alternatives" from the 0 Point Food List, including proteins, ingredients, instructions, nutritional information, serving size, and cooking time.

Food Item	Ingredients	Instructions	Nutritional Information	Serving Size	Cooking Time
Non-Fat Greek Yogurt	1 cup non-fat Greek yogurt	Scoop into a bowl or use as a base for smoothies or recipes.	100 calories, 10g protein, 5g carbs, 0g fat	1 cup	0 minutes
Skim Milk	1 cup skim milk	Pour directly into a glass or use in cooking	80 calories, 8g protein, 12g carbs, 0g fat	1 cup	0 minutes

		and baking.			
Unswe eetened Almon d Milk	1 cup unsweet ened almond milk	Shake before use. Can be consum ed as is or used in recipes.	30 calories, 1g protein, 1g carbs, 2.5g fat	1 cup	0 minutes
Non-Fa t Cottag e Cheese	1 cup non-fat cottage cheese	Use as a snack or add to salads and dishes.	80 calories, 11g protein, 4g carbs, 0g fat	1 cup	0 minutes
Non-Fa t Plain Yogurt	1 cup non-fat plain yogurt	Eat directly or mix with fruit and	100 calories, 9g protein, 12g	1 cup	0 minutes

		honey for added flavor.	carbs, 0g fat		
Soy Milk (Unsweetened)	1 cup unsweetened soy milk	Shake well before use. Consume as a beverage or use in cooking.	80 calories, 7g protein, 4g carbs, 4g fat	1 cup	0 minutes
Non-Fat Kefir	1 cup non-fat kefir	Drink directly or use in smoothies and dressings.	100 calories, 10g protein, 12g carbs, 0g fat	1 cup	0 minutes

Ricott a Cheese (Non-F at)	1 cup non-fat ricotta cheese	Use in cooking , baking, or as a topping .	300 calories, 28g protein, 12g carbs, 0g fat	1 cup	0 minutes
Non-Fa t Cream Cheese	2 tablesp oons non-fat cream cheese	Use as a spread or in cooking .	40 calories, 4g protein, 1g carbs, 1g fat	2 tablesp oons	0 minutes
Butter milk (Low-F at)	1 cup low-fat butter milk	Use in baking or as a drink.	100 calories, 8g protein, 12g carbs, 2g fat	1 cup	0 minutes
Almon d Milk Yogurt	1 cup unsweet ened	Enjoy as a snack	60 calories, 1g	1 cup	0 minutes

(Unswe etened)	almond milk yogurt	or mix with fruit.	protein, 4g carbs, 3g fat		
Goat Milk (Skim)	1 cup skim goat milk	Consu me as a beverag e or use in recipes.	120 calories, 8g protein, 11g carbs, 4g fat	1 cup	0 minutes
Cashe w Milk (Unswe etened)	1 cup unsweet ened cashew milk	Shake before drinkin g or use in cooking .	25 calories, 1g protein, 1g carbs, 2g fat	1 cup	0 minutes
Cocon ut Milk (Light)	1 cup light coconut milk	Use in recipes or as a beverag e.	45 calories, 1g protein, 3g	1 cup	0 minutes

			carbs, 3g fat		
Hemp Milk (Unsweetened)	1 cup unsweetened hemp milk	Shake well before drinking or use in cooking.	70 calories, 3g protein, 1g carbs, 5g fat	1 cup	0 minutes

This table provides a concise overview of the various dairy and dairy alternatives available on the 0 Point Food List, making it easy to understand how to incorporate these items into your diet while adhering to the guidelines.

Grains

Here's a detailed table on "Grains" as part of the food groups to eat in "The Complete 0 Point Food List." It includes 15 grain ingredients with their instructions, nutritional information, serving size, and cooking time.

Grain Ingredient	Instructions	Nutritional Information	Serving Size	Cooking Time
Quinoa	Rinse under cold water. Combine 1 cup quinoa with 2 cups water or broth in a pot. Bring to a boil, then	1 cup cooked: 222 calories, 8g protein, 39g carbs, 3.6g fat	1 cup cooked	20 minutes

	reduce heat, cover, and simmer for 15 minutes. Let it stand for 5 minutes before fluffing with a fork.			
Brown Rice	Rinse under cold water. Combine 1 cup brown rice with 2.5 cups water or broth in a pot. Bring	1 cup cooked: 215 calories, 5g protein, 45g carbs, 1.8g fat	1 cup cooked	50 minutes

	to a boil, then reduce heat, cover, and simmer for 45 minutes. Let it stand for 5 minutes before serving.			
Oats	Combine 1 cup oats with 2 cups water or milk in a pot. Bring to a boil, then reduce heat and simmer	1 cup cooked: 154 calories, 6g protein, 27g carbs, 3g fat	1 cup cooked	5 minutes

	for 5 minutes, stirring occasionally. For thicker oatmeal, cook for an additional 2-3 minutes.			
Barley	Rinse under cold water. Combine 1 cup barley with 3 cups water or broth in a pot. Bring to a boil,	1 cup cooked: 193 calories, 3.5g protein, 44g carbs, 0.6g fat	1 cup cooked	50-60 minutes

	then reduce heat, cover, and simmer for 45 minutes to 1 hour. Drain any excess liquid.			
Bulgur	Combine 1 cup bulgur with 1.5 cups boiling water. Cover and let it sit for 10 minutes. Fluff with a fork.	1 cup cooked: 151 calories, 5g protein, 34g carbs, 0.5g fat	1 cup cooked	10 minutes

Farro	Rinse under cold water. Combine 1 cup farro with 3 cups water or broth in a pot. Bring to a boil, then reduce heat, cover, and simmer for 30 minutes. Drain any excess liquid.	1 cup cooked: 170 calories, 6g protein, 35g carbs, 1g fat	1 cup cooked	30 minutes
Millet	Rinse under cold	1 cup cooked: 207	1 cup cooked	20 minutes

	water. Combine 1 cup millet with 2 cups water or broth in a pot. Bring to a boil, then reduce heat, cover, and simmer for 20 minutes. Let it stand for 5 minutes before fluffing with a fork.	calories, 6g protein, 41g carbs, 1.7g fat		

Buckwheat	Rinse under cold water. Combine 1 cup buckwheat groats with 2 cups water or broth in a pot. Bring to a boil, then reduce heat, cover, and simmer for 10-15 minutes. Let it stand for 5 minutes before serving.	1 cup cooked: 155 calories, 6g protein, 33g carbs, 1g fat	1 cup cooked	15 minutes

Rye Berries	Rinse under cold water. Combine 1 cup rye berries with 3 cups water or broth in a pot. Bring to a boil, then reduce heat, cover, and simmer for 1 hour. Drain any excess liquid.	1 cup cooked: 217 calories, 6g protein, 45g carbs, 1g fat	1 cup cooked	60 minutes
Amaranth	Rinse under	1 cup cooked:	1 cup cooked	20 minutes

	cold water. Combine 1 cup amaranth with 2.5 cups water or broth in a pot. Bring to a boil, then reduce heat, cover, and simmer for 20 minutes. Let it stand for 5 minutes before fluffing with a fork.	251 calories, 9g protein, 46g carbs, 4g fat		

| Teff | Rinse under cold water. Combine 1 cup teff with 3 cups water or broth in a pot. Bring to a boil, then reduce heat, cover, and simmer for 15 minutes. Let it stand for 5 minutes before serving. | 1 cup cooked: 255 calories, 10g protein, 50g carbs, 1.5g fat | 1 cup cooked | 15 minutes |

Freekeh	Rinse under cold water. Combine 1 cup freekeh with 2.5 cups water or broth in a pot. Bring to a boil, then reduce heat, cover, and simmer for 20-25 minutes. Drain any excess liquid.	1 cup cooked: 180 calories, 6g protein, 35g carbs, 1g fat	1 cup cooked	25 minutes
Couscous	Combine 1 cup	1 cup cooked:	1 cup cooked	5 minutes

	couscous with 1.5 cups boiling water. Cover and let it sit for 5 minutes. Fluff with a fork before serving.	176 calories, 6g protein, 36g carbs, 0.3g fat		
Spelt	Rinse under cold water. Combine 1 cup spelt with 2.5 cups water or broth in a pot. Bring to a boil,	1 cup cooked: 246 calories, 10g protein, 44g carbs, 1.5g fat	1 cup cooked	30 minutes

	then reduce heat, cover, and simmer for 30 minutes. Drain any excess liquid.			
Kamut	Rinse under cold water. Combine 1 cup kamut with 3 cups water or broth in a pot. Bring to a boil, then reduce	1 cup cooked: 251 calories, 10g protein, 55g carbs, 2g fat	1 cup cooked	60 minutes

	heat, cover, and simmer for 1 hour. Drain any excess liquid.			

This table provides an overview of various grains you can incorporate into your diet, along with cooking instructions, nutritional values, serving sizes, and approximate cooking times.

Chapter 2: Foods to Avoid

High-Calorie Vegetables

Here's a detailed table on "High-Calorie Vegetables" as part of the foods to avoid in relation to "The Complete 0 Point Food List," including the types of vegetables and reasons for avoiding them.

High-Calorie Vegetable	Calories per 1 Cup Cooked	Reason to Avoid
Avocado	234 calories	Avocado is high in calories and fats, which can contribute significantly to daily caloric intake. While it provides healthy fats, its high caloric density can make it difficult to manage portion sizes and meet weight loss goals.

Corn	143 calories	Corn is high in carbohydrates and calories compared to many other vegetables. It can lead to excess calorie consumption, making it harder to control weight if not eaten in moderation.
Sweet Potatoes	180 calories	Sweet potatoes are nutrient-dense but also high in calories and carbohydrates. Their caloric density can add up quickly, which might not align with a low-calorie eating plan.
Potatoes	130 calories	Potatoes, especially when prepared

		with added fats, can be high in calories. They also have a high glycemic index, which can affect blood sugar levels and overall calorie control.
Butternut Squash	82 calories	While not excessively high in calories, butternut squash has more calories than many other non-starchy vegetables. It should be eaten in moderation to avoid excess calorie intake.
Pumpkin	49 calories	Pumpkin is relatively high in calories compared to non-starchy vegetables.

		Though nutritious, consuming it in large amounts can impact caloric goals.
Beets	59 calories	Beets are high in natural sugars and calories compared to many other vegetables. Their calorie content can add up quickly, impacting overall caloric control.
Carrots	55 calories	Carrots, while nutritious, are higher in calories than other non-starchy vegetables. Excessive consumption can affect calorie balance.

Peas	117 calories	Peas are relatively high in calories and carbohydrates compared to other vegetables. They should be eaten in moderation to maintain caloric control.
Artichokes	60 calories	Artichokes have more calories than many other vegetables. Although they are high in fiber and nutrients, their caloric density can impact weight management if consumed in large quantities.
Parsnips	100 calories	Parsnips are higher in calories and carbohydrates compared to many

		non-starchy vegetables. They can contribute to excess calorie intake if not moderated.
Yams	157 calories	Yams are high in calories and carbohydrates. Their caloric density can make it challenging to stay within a low-calorie eating plan.
Jicama	49 calories	While relatively low in calories, jicama is still higher in calories compared to other non-starchy vegetables and should be consumed in moderation.

Plantains	122 calories	Plantains are high in calories and carbohydrates. Their caloric content can quickly add up, affecting overall calorie management.
Kohlrabi	36 calories	Although lower in calories compared to others on this list, kohlrabi has more calories than many non-starchy vegetables and should be consumed in reasonable amounts.

This table provides an overview of high-calorie vegetables and the reasons to limit or avoid them when following a 0 point food plan. These vegetables, while nutritious, have higher caloric densities which can interfere with weight management goals if consumed in large quantities.

Fruits with Added Sugars

Here is a detailed table about "Fruits with Added Sugars" as foods to avoid in relation to "The Complete 0 Point Food List," including specific fruits with added sugars and reasons why they should be avoided:

Fruit with Added Sugars	Reason to Avoid	Typical Sugar Content	Common Forms
Dried Fruits (e.g., Raisins, Dates)	High sugar content due to concentration during drying, which increases calorie density and can lead to excessive sugar intake.	1 cup of raisins: approximatel y 115 grams of sugar	Raisins, dates, apricots, figs
Fruit Juices (e.g.,	Often contains	8 oz of orange juice:	Bottled orange juice,

Orange Juice, Apple Juice)	added sugars and lacks the fiber found in whole fruits, leading to rapid sugar absorption and increased calorie intake.	approximatel y 22 grams of sugar	apple juice, grape juice
Canned Fruits in Syrup (e.g., Peaches, Pineapples)	Packed in sugary syrup, which significantly increases the sugar content and overall calorie count.	1 cup of canned peaches in syrup: approximatel y 30 grams of sugar	Canned peaches, pineapples, pears
Frozen Fruits with Added Sugars (e.g., Frozen Berries, Mangoes)	Sugar is added to enhance flavor and preservation, leading to higher sugar	1 cup of frozen strawberries with added sugar: approximatel	Frozen strawberries, mango chunks, mixed fruit blends

	content compared to fresh or unsweetened frozen fruits.	y 20 grams of sugar	
Fruit-flavored Yogurts (e.g., Strawberry, Blueberry Yogurt)	Contains added sugars to enhance fruit flavor, contributing to excess sugar intake and potential weight gain.	6 oz of strawberry yogurt: approximately 20 grams of sugar	Flavored yogurts, fruit-on-the-bottom yogurts
Smoothies with Added Sweeteners (e.g., Store-bought Smoothies)	May contain added syrups or sweetened fruit concentrates, which increases sugar levels and caloric content.	16 oz store-bought smoothie: approximately 40 grams of sugar	Bottled fruit smoothies, pre-made smoothie mixes

Fruit Bars (e.g., Fruit and Nut Bars, Fruit Roll-ups)	Often include added sugars or high-fructose corn syrup, making them high in sugar and calories.	1 fruit bar: approximatel y 15 grams of sugar	Fruit snacks, fruit leather, energy bars
Flavored Fruit Drinks (e.g., Fruit Punch, Flavored Water)	Typically contain high levels of added sugars or sweeteners, contributing to excess calorie and sugar intake.	12 oz fruit punch: approximatel y 30 grams of sugar	Fruit punch, flavored waters with fruit essence
Preserves and Jams (e.g., Strawberry Jam, Grape Jelly)	High in added sugars used to enhance flavor and preserve the	1 tablespoon of strawberry jam: approximatel y 10 grams of sugar	Fruit preserves, jelly, marmalade

	fruit, resulting in high sugar content.		
Sweetened Applesauce	Added sugars increase the calorie content and sugar intake, making it less beneficial than unsweetened applesauce.	1 cup of sweetened applesauce: approximatel y 24 grams of sugar	Sweetened applesauce, fruit sauces

Avoiding fruits with added sugars helps maintain lower calorie and sugar intake, supports better blood sugar control, and promotes overall health. These processed fruits and products can contribute to weight gain and other health issues due to their high sugar content and lack of beneficial fiber. Opting for fresh, whole fruits without added sugars ensures you receive the full nutritional benefits while keeping your sugar intake in check.

Processed Proteins

Here is a detailed table about "Processed Proteins" under the section of foods to avoid in relation to "The Complete 0 Point Food List," including various types of processed proteins and reasons for their exclusion from a healthy eating plan.

Processed Protein	Description	Reasons to Avoid
Bacon	Cured and smoked pork belly, typically high in fat and sodium.	High in saturated fats and cholesterol, contributing to heart disease. It also contains added nitrates and preservatives that may have negative health effects.
Sausages	Processed meat encased in a casing, often made from pork, beef, or poultry.	Often high in saturated fats, sodium, and preservatives like nitrates and nitrites, which are

		linked to increased risk of cancer and cardiovascular diseases.
Hot Dogs	Pre-cooked or cured sausages made from beef, pork, or poultry.	Contains high levels of sodium, unhealthy fats, and preservatives. Frequent consumption has been associated with an increased risk of heart disease and cancer.
Deli Meats	Processed meats such as ham, turkey, or roast beef used in sandwiches.	Typically high in sodium, preservatives, and unhealthy fats. These factors can contribute to hypertension, cardiovascular diseases, and other health issues.

Pepperoni	Spicy, cured sausage made from beef and pork, often used on pizza.	Contains high levels of saturated fats, sodium, and preservatives. Regular consumption may increase the risk of heart disease and other chronic conditions.
Salami	Fermented and cured sausage made from pork, beef, or other meats.	High in saturated fats, sodium, and preservatives. It has been linked to negative health effects including heart disease and cancer.
Corned Beef	Salt-cured beef, often used in sandwiches and stews.	High in sodium and saturated fats. Excessive consumption can lead to increased risk of hypertension,

		heart disease, and other health problems.
Chicken Nuggets	Breaded and deep-fried pieces of chicken.	Often contains unhealthy fats, sodium, and preservatives. The frying process adds extra calories and unhealthy fats, which can contribute to weight gain and cardiovascular issues.
Spam	Canned meat product made from pork shoulder and ham.	High in sodium, fat, and preservatives. Consuming spam regularly can contribute to hypertension, cardiovascular diseases, and obesity.

Pastrami	Cured and smoked beef, typically used in sandwiches.	High in sodium, saturated fats, and preservatives. Excessive consumption is associated with negative health outcomes including heart disease and cancer.
Potted Meat	Canned meat product, often made from beef or pork.	Contains high levels of sodium, fat, and preservatives. Regular consumption can have adverse effects on cardiovascular health and overall well-being.
Liverwurst	Spreadable sausage made from liver and other meats.	High in fat, sodium, and cholesterol. Regular consumption can

		contribute to health issues such as heart disease and high blood pressure.
Beef Jerky	Dried and salted strips of beef.	Often high in sodium and preservatives. The drying process concentrates these elements, which can have negative health effects when consumed in large quantities.
Vienna Sausages	Canned sausages made from pork and beef.	High in sodium, unhealthy fats, and preservatives. Frequent consumption can lead to increased risk of hypertension and cardiovascular diseases.

Bologna	Processed meat product made from finely ground beef, pork, or poultry.	Contains high amounts of sodium, fat, and preservatives. Regular consumption can increase the risk of cardiovascular diseases and other health issues.

This table outlines various processed proteins to avoid and explains why they should be excluded from a healthy eating plan, emphasizing the negative health impacts of these foods.

High-Fat Dairy Products

Here is a detailed table about "High-Fat Dairy Products" as foods to avoid in relation to "The Complete 0 Point Food List." It includes various high-fat dairy products and reasons why they should be avoided:

High-Fat Dairy Product	Reason to Avoid
Whole Milk	Whole milk contains a high amount of saturated fat and calories compared to skim or low-fat milk. Consuming it regularly can contribute to weight gain and increase your risk of heart disease.
Heavy Cream	Heavy cream is rich in saturated fats and calories, which can lead to increased cholesterol levels and weight gain. It's often used in cooking and baking, making it easy to consume in large quantities.

Full-Fat Cheese	Full-fat cheeses such as cheddar, mozzarella, and Swiss are high in saturated fats and calories. Frequent consumption can contribute to cardiovascular issues and excessive calorie intake.
Butter	Butter is high in saturated fat and calories. Using it in cooking or as a spread can significantly increase your daily fat intake, which may lead to weight gain and health problems.
Cream Cheese	Cream cheese is high in fat and calories, making it a less healthy choice for spreads and dips. Its high fat content can contribute to higher cholesterol levels and weight gain.
Whipped Cream	Whipped cream, often used as a topping or in desserts, is high in saturated fat and

	sugar. Its calorie density can lead to weight gain and increased risk of metabolic issues.
Clotted Cream	Clotted cream is extremely high in saturated fat and calories. It is often used in high-calorie desserts and can significantly contribute to excessive fat and calorie intake.
Double Cream	Double cream has a high fat content, particularly saturated fat, which can negatively affect heart health and contribute to weight gain when consumed frequently.
Cream-Based Sauces	Sauces made with heavy cream, such as Alfredo or creamy gravies, are high in saturated fats and calories. They can significantly increase the caloric and fat content of meals.

Full-Fat Greek Yogurt	While Greek yogurt can be a healthy choice, full-fat versions are high in saturated fat and calories. Choosing non-fat or low-fat options is preferable for managing calorie and fat intake.
Ice Cream	Ice cream is high in both saturated fats and added sugars, contributing to excessive calorie intake and potential weight gain. It can also lead to blood sugar spikes.
Cheese Curds	Cheese curds are high in saturated fat and calories. Eating them in large amounts can contribute to excessive calorie and fat consumption, negatively impacting heart health.
Mascarpone Cheese	Mascarpone cheese is rich in fat and calories. It is often used in desserts, which can

	add significant calories and unhealthy fats to your diet.
Ricotta Cheese (Whole Milk)	Whole milk ricotta cheese is high in fat and calories. It can add unnecessary calories and saturated fats to your diet, leading to weight gain and other health issues.

High-fat dairy products should be avoided or consumed in moderation due to their high saturated fat content and calorie density. Regular intake of these products can lead to weight gain, increased cholesterol levels, and higher risk of heart disease. Opting for lower-fat or non-dairy alternatives can help maintain a healthier diet and support overall well-being.

Refined Grains and Sugars

Here's a detailed table on "Refined Grains and Sugars" as foods to avoid in relation to "The Complete 0 Point Food List." The table includes types of refined grains and sugars, reasons to avoid them, and their potential impact on health.

Refined Grain/Sugar	Why You Should Avoid It	Potential Impact on Health
White Bread	Made from highly processed flour, which lacks fiber and nutrients. Often contains added sugars and preservatives.	Contributes to weight gain, increases blood sugar levels, and can lead to insulin resistance.
White Rice	Stripped of its bran and germ during processing, resulting in a loss of fiber and nutrients.	Can cause spikes in blood sugar and contribute to poor digestive health.
Pastries	Typically made with refined flour	High in empty calories, which can

	and high amounts of sugar and fat.	lead to weight gain and metabolic issues.
Cookies	Made from refined flour and sugar, with added fats and preservatives.	Can lead to increased cravings, weight gain, and higher risk of chronic diseases.
Cakes	Often contain refined flour, sugars, and unhealthy fats.	Can cause rapid blood sugar spikes and contribute to overall poor diet quality.
Cereals (Sugary)	Usually made with refined grains and added sugars. Often lacks essential nutrients.	Can lead to poor blood sugar control and increased risk of diabetes and heart disease.
Pasta (Regular)	Made from refined wheat flour, which is low in fiber and nutrients.	Can contribute to weight gain and metabolic issues,

		such as insulin resistance.
Bagels	Typically made with refined flour and high in calories.	Can lead to increased hunger and poor dietary quality due to low fiber content.
Crackers (Regular)	Often made with refined grains and added sugars or fats.	Can contribute to weight gain and poor blood sugar control.
White Flour	Lacks fiber and nutrients due to processing.	Can lead to increased risk of digestive issues and chronic diseases.
Instant Oatmeal	Often contains added sugars and is made from processed oats.	Can cause spikes in blood sugar and lead to increased cravings for unhealthy foods.

Energy Bars (Sugary)	Frequently made with refined grains and sugars.	Often high in empty calories and can contribute to weight gain and poor energy levels.
Tortillas (White)	Typically made from refined flour, lacking essential nutrients and fiber.	Can lead to poor blood sugar control and contribute to weight gain.
Pop-Tarts	Made with refined flour and high amounts of sugar and fats.	Can cause rapid blood sugar spikes and contribute to overall poor dietary quality.
Sweetened Yogurts	Often contain added sugars and are made with low-fat or processed ingredients.	Can contribute to increased calorie intake and poor metabolic health.

Avoiding refined grains and sugars is crucial for maintaining balanced nutrition and overall health. These foods are often stripped of essential nutrients and fiber during processing, leading to quick spikes in blood sugar and increased hunger, which can contribute to weight gain and various health issues. By opting for whole grains and natural sources of sweetness, you can better manage your weight and support your long-term well-being.

Chapter 3: Sample Meal Plans

Breakfast: Veggie-Packed Egg White Omelet

- Ingredients:
  - 1 cup egg whites
  - 1/2 cup diced bell peppers
  - 1/2 cup spinach
  - 1/4 cup diced onions
  - 1/4 cup mushrooms
  - 1/4 cup diced tomatoes
  - Salt and pepper to taste

- Instructions:
  1. Heat a non-stick skillet over medium heat.
  2. Add onions and mushrooms, and sauté for 3-4 minutes until softened.
  3. Add bell peppers, spinach, and tomatoes, and cook for an additional 2 minutes.
  4. Pour egg whites over the vegetables and cook until set, about 4-5 minutes.
  5. Fold the omelet in half and serve.

- Nutritional Information:
  - Calories: 120

- Protein: 20g
- Carbs: 10g
- Fat: 0g

- **Serving Size:** 1 omelet

- **Cooking Time:** 10 minutes

Lunch: Quinoa and Black Bean Salad

- **Ingredients:**
  - 1 cup cooked quinoa
  - 1/2 cup black beans, rinsed and drained
  - 1/2 cup corn kernels
  - 1/2 cup cherry tomatoes, halved
  - 1/4 cup chopped cilantro
  - Juice of 1 lime
  - Salt and pepper to taste

- **Instructions:**
  1. In a large bowl, combine quinoa, black beans, corn, cherry tomatoes, and cilantro.
  2. Toss with lime juice, salt, and pepper.
  3. Chill for at least 30 minutes before serving.

- **Nutritional Information:**

- Calories: 250
- Protein: 9g
- Carbs: 45g
- Fat: 2g

- **Serving Size:** 1 cup

- **Cooking Time:** 10 minutes (plus 30 minutes chilling time)

Dinner: Baked Salmon with Steamed Broccoli

- **Ingredients:**
  - 1 6-ounce salmon fillet
  - 1 tablespoon lemon juice
  - 1 teaspoon dried dill
  - 1 cup broccoli florets
  - Salt and pepper to taste

- **Instructions:**
  1. Preheat oven to 375°F (190°C).
  2. Place salmon on a baking sheet lined with parchment paper. Drizzle with lemon juice and sprinkle with dill, salt, and pepper.
  3. Bake for 15-20 minutes, or until salmon flakes easily with a fork.
  4. Steam broccoli florets for 5-7 minutes until tender.

- **Nutritional Information:**
  - Calories: 300
  - Protein: 30g
  - Carbs: 10g
  - Fat: 15g

- **Serving Size:** 1 fillet with 1 cup broccoli

- **Cooking Time:** 20 minutes

Snacks: Fresh Fruit and Air-Popped Popcorn

- **Ingredients:**
  - 1 medium apple
  - 1 cup air-popped popcorn

- **Instructions:**
  1. Slice the apple into wedges.
  2. Serve with air-popped popcorn.

- **Nutritional Information:**
  - Calories: 180
  - Protein: 2g
  - Carbs: 45g

- Fat: 1g

- **Serving Size:** 1 apple and 1 cup popcorn

- **Cooking Time:** 5 minutes (for slicing apple and popping popcorn)

Conclusion

As you conclude your journey through "The Complete 0 Point Food List," it's clear that integrating these foods into your daily routine offers a practical and sustainable approach to healthy eating. By focusing on foods that have zero points, you simplify meal planning and reduce the complexity often associated with weight management and nutritional balance. This approach not only supports weight loss but also promotes overall well-being by emphasizing nutrient-dense options.

The 0 point foods highlighted in the guide are carefully selected for their health benefits, including vegetables, fruits, and lean proteins. These foods are rich in essential nutrients while being low in calories, allowing you to eat satisfying portions without compromising your dietary goals. Incorporating these foods can help manage hunger and cravings, making it easier to stick to a healthy eating plan.

The practical advice offered within the guide, such as sample meal plans and recipes, provides a structured framework to get started. By following these examples, you can quickly adapt to using 0 point foods in your meals, ensuring variety and flavor while maintaining a focus on nutrition. The flexibility of these meal plans allows you to customize them according to your preferences and lifestyle.

Understanding which foods to avoid is equally important. Refined grains and sugars, while often appealing, can derail your progress by contributing empty calories and affecting blood sugar levels. By steering clear of these items and focusing on whole, unprocessed foods, you enhance your dietary quality and support long-term health goals.

The detailed information on cooking times and nutritional content provided in the guide helps you make informed decisions and optimize meal preparation. This knowledge empowers you to create meals that are both delicious and aligned with your health objectives. Proper planning and preparation ensure that you can maintain your commitment to a healthy lifestyle with ease.

Remember that the journey to better health is a gradual process, and using this guide as a tool can provide ongoing support. The principles and strategies outlined in the guide are designed to be sustainable and adaptable, allowing you to make lasting changes in your eating habits. Consistency and mindfulness in choosing 0 point foods will contribute significantly to achieving and maintaining your health goals.

In summary, "The Complete 0 Point Food List" offers a comprehensive approach to healthier eating by focusing on nutrient-rich, zero-point foods. Embracing the guidance and recommendations provided will help you make informed choices, stay on track with your dietary goals, and ultimately lead to a healthier, more balanced lifestyle. The principles outlined in the guide are not just about what you eat but about fostering a positive relationship with food and making choices that support your overall well-being.

Printed in Great Britain
by Amazon

46689198R00056